100 Self-Care Activities for Men

Edgar Wise

FREE EBOOK

SIGN UP TO MY MAILING LIST TO GET A FREE EBOOK

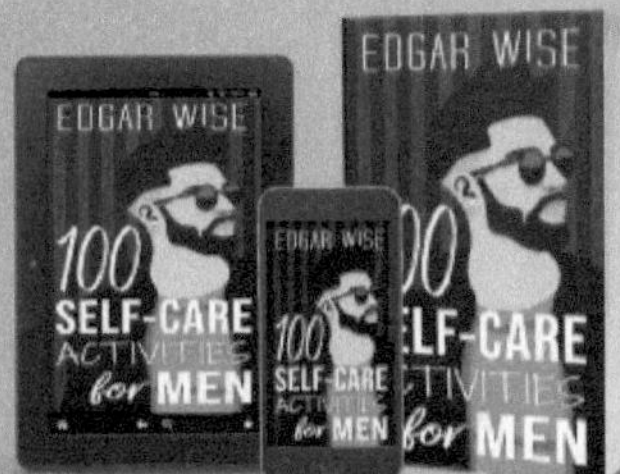

More freebies...

 Receive weekly self-improvement tips.

 Get advanced readers' copy of my books for FREE!

 Get a chance to download audiobooks for FREE!

 Get a chance to win paperback giveaways.

 And more!

www.edgarwise.com

Contents

Introduction   2

100 Self-Care Activities for Men   6

Conclusion   42

Leaving a Review   46

Introduction

Self-care is truly a simple thing. Despite this, the majority of men have never been taught about self-care, nor do they realize how critical it is for their emotional and mental well-being. It is important to remember that for most of you, the way you were raised has a lot to do with why you may or may not be good at treating yourself lovingly and respectfully. With that said, dealing with self-care doesn't have to be complex or expensive. You can take some time for yourself by doing simple things such as taking bubble baths, meditating, reading to relax, and playing video games. The most important thing with self-care is allowing yourself the time and space you need to indulge in your favorite hobbies without feeling guilty about neglecting other responsibilities or relationships you may have.

If you are not good at caring for yourself first, how will you ever learn the skills to care for others? How can you be a good partner, father, brother, or son if you have never taken the time to care for yourself?

Self-care is not selfish. Neglecting your needs will only make you feel like less of a man because it makes you feel like you are not your best self. Caring for others only happens when you have first cared for yourself. The more attention you give yourself, the more you will have to share with those around you: friends, family, and loved ones. It is important to remember that everyone comes into your life for a reason. However, this may be challenging to understand at times until much later on after they have left your life. So, always learn from the relationships in your life as each one will teach you something about yourself.

Many times, you don't know how to take care of yourself because you have had so little practice doing it. If this is the case for you, then it is recommended that you begin by identifying what makes you happy and then create some time in your schedule to do those things. Today may be the only chance you have to take some time out of your busy and stressful life for yourself. Life can often feel like it's too much, and sometimes you need to give yourself permission to slow down, sit back and relax, and make your needs a priority. Taking care of yourself is giving orders from within that say, "I am important, I need to be taken care of, and I deserve relaxation time."

There is no right or wrong way to go about doing self-care because only you would know how much time you have to invest in yourself. If you think that taking a break from the world for an hour will help you lower your stress level, then do it. Just remove yourself from your surroundings and find some space. You will feel better afterward as long as you permit yourself to relax. Do not let guilt or judgment creep back into your mind if you get interrupted during this time because things happen without notice, such as mobile phones ringing, people texting, or just someone needing help with something. This doesn't mean that what you're doing is wrong; it just means that you have a busy life and others depend on you. Make time in your day for your self-care because you deserve it so that you can then be of service to those around you.

So, it is time to start treating yourself with the love and respect that you deserve. It is fine to have needs, wants, and desires. Nurturing your mind and body is an important part of self-care.

Hopefully, this short book can inspire any man to get started taking care of himself. Likewise, may these suggestions serve as encouragement for all not to wait until it's too late.

100 Self-Care Activities for Men

1. Make it a habit to wake up early.

Everyone knows that early risers are more effective and productive. Try to start your day with fresh air and exercise. This will help you be more awake, clear-headed, and happier throughout the day, both mentally and physically. Most people feel better after a good night's sleep as well, so that's another reason to wake up early in most cases.

2. Eat breakfast every morning.

Breakfast is the most important meal of the day. This doesn't have to be a big meal, but just something small like some fruit or maybe a slice of toast with peanut butter on it. Eating breakfast every morning helps jumpstart your metabolism in the morning, preventing you from feeling sluggish and tired. It will help keep your energy levels up which is very important before participating in any type of exercise.

3. Take a cold shower.

It's been said that taking a cold shower can help a person calm down and relieve stress. It may sound counterintuitive, but in fact, your heart rate and blood pressure actually drop when you first step into the cold water. In addition, it forces you to focus solely on the sensation of the water hitting your skin because there isn't time for your mind to wander elsewhere.

4. Exercise outside if possible at least once per day.

If you live near a beach or forest, go there to be around trees and breathe in the fresher air. If not, just find a park or some open land to run around. It's great for your mind and body to take in the outdoors first thing in the morning, if possible.

5. Make sure to take your vitamins daily.

These are essential substances to your well-being that can help you prevent getting sick. These can boost your immune system and make sure you have energy for the day. You're going to need these nutrients for your physical and brain activities.

6. Wash your hands frequently during the day.

It sounds simple enough, but keeping your hands clean is one of the best ways to ward off disease-causing bacteria from invading and infecting you. Using soap is best, but if you can't find any, just use water. Also, try to avoid touching your face with dirty hands, as this is one of the most common ways germs spread from person to person.

7. Drink at least 2 liters of clean, freshwater each day.

It keeps you hydrated which is essential for the proper functioning of every system in your body. If you like, you can try adding lemon juice to your water with some honey. This makes it taste better and if you drink enough of this throughout the day, you'll find that your immune system will function better too.

8. Wash all of your clothes every week at the very least.

If possible, wash them in hot water – especially underwear and socks. This kills off any bacteria or germs. One tip is that you can add vinegar to your laundry as well which helps prevent mold and sour odors in clothing from growing over time. White vinegar's acidic nature makes it an excellent whitener and brightener for dirty white and colored clothing.

9. Wash all your bed sheets, blankets, and pillowcases every other week in hot water.

This will help remove any bacteria or germs that may have gotten on them. It is also a good idea to toss out your pillows every few years since they get compressed over time. Replacing them helps prevent mold from growing inside of them which can be unhealthy.

10. Use natural products for your hygiene needs.

Most common personal hygiene items such as toothpaste, soap, shampoo, conditioner, and deodorant, among others, that are found in most homes these days contain toxic chemicals that can cause harm to the body and your health over time if used too much. This is why it is recommended to use natural versions of all of these. There are many companies that offer green versions of each item listed above so it shouldn't be too hard to find replacements for everything you normally use.

11. Get plenty of rest throughout the week.

It is recommended to go to bed early and catch up on sleep whenever you can during the day. It's easy for people who work during the week to become overly stressed out with their jobs which in turn causes insomnia or simply sleeping too little. Either way, it's bad for your health and leads to a wide range of problems down the road – don't let this happen. Get rest when you can but don't forget about working hard at everything that you do.

12. Listen to some relaxing music with quality headphones before going to bed every night.

You can listen to classical music, jazz, or anything slow and mellow. It is a proven fact that this helps you sleep faster. You can increase the quality of sleep with this small step.

13. Go outside every day for at least 30 minutes (preferably an hour or longer).

There's something about fresh air that just makes you feel better. Take in as many deep breaths as possible when outside and try not to focus on anything negative that may be happening around you. Spending time outside also helps improve circulation, increases oxygen flow throughout the body, increases the immune system's overall strength and so much more.

14. Take a short walk outside or around your house every day during breaks.

You may do this in between studying, working, or even playing games. It's okay to take small walks so long as you don't go too far from home and lose focus on what you are currently doing. Walking helps increase circulation, helps strengthen muscles, and improves brain function. It's great for staying healthy overall. And if you have a dog, then try taking him with you when doing this in order to get some exercise since walking with a pet can be quite fun and beneficial if done right.

15. Strike up a positive conversation with a friend or a stranger no matter how much you don't want to or feel like it.

There's something about talking with others that just makes everything in your life feel better. Make sure that the person is someone who's genuinely friendly and who seems to care about what you do and the activities you are involved in. Perhaps, they can also give suggestions and helpful tips to your pursuits.

16. 'Smile' when speaking to others.

Approach people, even strangers with confidence, and make sure to be honest as well as respectful whenever talking to someone new. Do not say something that is too short. At least try to show some interest in talking with them.

17. Use your vacation time.

Men are notorious for taking less vacation than they are actually allotted. When you get busy, it can be hard to take a break from your daily grind. But, that's exactly what needs to happen when you're feeling stressed or overwhelmed by the expectations of your job and life in general. Even if it's just an extra day or weekend once in a while, getting away truly does help you feel refreshed and ready to tackle whatever challenges that may come next.

18. Build something with your hands.

Whether you are an avid woodworker or have never held a hammer in your life, getting into the zone and producing some crafty work can be a good way to let yourself go. If you don't want to spend money on tools, there are plenty of tutorials online for DIY projects using things like toothpicks and binder clips.

19. Organize your workspace.

Put away all the papers, pens, and notebooks you currently have strewn across your desk. Clean off what you can and organize it into different bins or folders. This gives the appearance of an organized workspace and will motivate you to stay organized.

20. Make sure to have plenty of things to do with your time while at home, work, or school.

Having too much free time may cause you more stress than you'd think. Even if you're able to take a break from work or school and relax for a little while, then it's often best not to have so much "free" time as this can eventually lead to nothing but boredom which tends to cause even more problems. Try keeping busy, even on your days off, by doing chores around the house and doing some light exercises.

21. Buy yourself small gifts that make you happy.

You may do this whenever you're having down periods or are feeling low about something. If it's not too expensive, then maybe get something as simple as an ice cream cone from your favorite shop or ice cream truck, and it is even better if it's summertime.

22. Get the current issues of men's fashion and lifestyle magazines.

Get inspired by reading through the profiles of refined men around the world. Let their stories inspire you to cultivate a refined lifestyle of your own. Think about what you actually want out of life, and then go do it.

23. Play video games.

Video games have been around for decades, and many people try to restrict game time in order to use that extra hour as "me" time. But playing video games is actually a great way to take care of yourself because it allows you to block out everything else—there's no need to be responsible or think ahead when the only thing you should be doing is concentrating on your game.

24. Watch a movie that makes you feel happy, hopeful, and proud of yourself for being alive.

Just make sure not to watch anything too sad or upsetting during your self-care time because that will get in the way of relaxing. If you just can't help it, then maybe try watching something with an uplifting ending so that you're left feeling good about life once again. Also, this is a great excuse to buy or rent some new movies from the video store or online if you haven't got any new ones to watch.

25. Listen to your favorite songs while dancing around the room for as long as you possibly can.

Try to get into the lyrics of the song and sing along at parts that you like, even if you're not a good singer. This is when music truly becomes alive. Don't worry about being messy or silly because it's just for fun. In fact, try putting on some goofy clothing too just so that you can be extra silly and have even more fun with yourself in your own little world of happiness. As an added bonus, make sure there are no witnesses around when doing these things because nobody needs to see how hilarious grown men can be.

26. Cook your favorite dish.

It could be a soup, a vegetable, or meat. It is the dish that you enjoy the most. But this time, do it in a way that is very different from how you normally would. Be aware of all your senses and focus as you cook. Then, enjoy every bite.

27. Bake a cake or pastry.

You may find a good recipe while watching TV. Depending on what you choose to bake, cupcake tins and cake pans may be needed. Serve it for dessert; decorate with colored sprinkles if you wish.

28. Try cooking a dish you haven't done before.

Maybe there's a recipe you've been wanting to try. Create a dish from scratch, or use recipes that you can find online. Either way, see what happens when you make your own meal. You might find the process fun and rewarding, or perhaps you'll see how easy it is to make mistakes when preparing a recipe.

29. Get a massage (or give one).

A great way to get rid of all the built-up tension or stress in your body is to have a nice relaxing rubdown. After all, what's better than having someone else scrub away at all the knots you have going on deep inside your muscles? You don't need to hire anyone for this. You can also ask or beg your partner, relatives, or close friends to give you a massage when they're free.

30. Go outside by yourself and stare at birds/clouds/trees.

This might sound weird but go ahead and try it. When you're out there alone staring aimlessly at nature, you will clear your mind of all the useless thoughts that plague your head on a regular basis. When you're out in nature, your mind eventually quiets down and begins to relax. Eventually, you will realize how small you are in relation to everything.

31. Paint your room.

This one may sound a bit odd, but it's surprisingly effective. There's something about getting out the paint and doing some art that can make you feel like you are actually accomplishing something, even if it is just painting your room. It also helps relieve stress.

32. Buy exercise equipment or items and actually use them.

Working out is a great way to let off some steam. If you're not the kind of guy who likes to work out in public, then it's always good to buy your own stuff so that you can do it whenever and wherever you want. It is recommended to get some resistance bands. They're cheap, easy to carry around and take up very little space in your homes which means you'll feel less likely to just leave them lying around unused once you get home from the store (which is usually what happens). You may also want to consider buying more expensive items like a treadmill, upright bike, weights, or a bench press.

33. Set up a meditation area in your house.

For some reason, many guys feel awkward sitting around and doing nothing so they are forced to go out just to get away from home for a while to avoid feeling stuck. However, you can avoid this by creating an entire meditation corner or area in your home that's free of distractions. This way you can sit there any time and do nothing if you want without having to leave the comfort of your own home.

34. Get rid of all distracting electronic devices from your bedroom.

It is highly recommended to try removing smartphones, laptops, and television sets, among others in your bedroom. All electronic devices will hinder your ability to sleep smoothly especially if you enjoy watching TV before going to bed. They make your body produce excess amounts of cortisol which is not good for your mental or physical health. Getting rid of these devices might be a big step so you can focus on your well-being without any distractions.

35. Read non-fiction books related to getting fit and healthy.

It seems like many guys simply don't know what's possible when it comes to being healthy or more ripped or muscular. The truth is that you can be anything from average-looking to ridiculously jacked depending on your genetics, diet, and training routine. Reading books will help clear away some misconceptions you might have about what's possible for yourself physically while also giving you ideas for how exactly you want to look at your maximum genetic potential.

36. Bike or walk to school/work instead of driving.

Instead of driving, why not ride a bike or walk especially when your school or workplace is just nearby? In addition to exercising, you'll also be getting a little extra cardio in your life as well, which is always good for you. On top of that, it gives you an opportunity to enjoy the fresh air and beautiful scenery while doing something healthy which can be very uplifting especially if you're a person who feels trapped and surrounded by concrete walls at times.

37. Go on a hike or go camping for the weekend.

Pack up some nice meat, or whatever meal plan that suits your needs. Get out there with friends and family while learning how to appreciate nature and your surroundings. Both hiking and camping require you to bring your own food which means you'll probably cook more. Doing this will allow you to try new things while not breaking the bank in the process. That said, it is recommended to invest in a small portable stove because it can be very handy when you're cooking with friends on a budget.

38. Get in touch with your local gym or community center.

There is a good chance they offer day passes that'll allow you to work out in their facilities for a low price. If not then at least, they might be able to point or recommend somewhere nearby that offers affordable prices, or will even pay for an entire month if you mention you're interested in signing up.

39. Go to yard sales or thrift shops.

People are always looking to get rid of stuff they don't need anymore so if you're able to find something useful for a really cheap price, then it might be worth taking advantage of. There's a good chance you'll find some very useful things like weights, exercise tapes or videos, etc. Just be careful when purchasing anything used because you never know what the condition is until after you've bought it and that can lead to lots of wasted money or time.

40. Start a garden even in little spaces.

This one is easy. Gardening is a great hobby and is healthy for you. Fresh vegetables, herbs, and even ornamental plants don't require a lot of room to grow. You don't even need a garden bed to get started. You can grow plants in little spaces if you have a container, water, and the sunlight. You can even embellish your windowsill with cacti and succulents.

41. Use the library during your search for free things to do.

Take full advantage of local libraries because they offer all sorts of useful resources. You can start using this place as a source for study materials, and then try branching out into audiobooks, e-books, films, videos, etc. This is another thing that will end up saving you plenty of cash in the long run.

42. Don't consume too much caffeine.

This is an unnecessary expense that will end up leaving you feeling jittery. If you've been using coffee as an excuse to snooze a few times, then think about how much sleep is worth in terms of how much you're willing to spend to get those few extra minutes.

43. Consider setting up an online forum regarding healthy living.

Everyone, including family and friends, can contribute their own thoughts, ideas, and suggestions on this virtual forum. It is also a great way to meet new friends as well. Doing something like this is an interesting route to go down at times because camaraderie is always good. Plus, if done correctly, it'll help out others as well.

44. Try living without a credit card for at least one month.

Don't make any impulse purchases either, because this is a good way to prove how much you really need it in your life. Also, if you do end up using it, then try setting some sort of limit for yourself before leaving the store, so that you won't overspend by accident.

45. Try eating out less by making your own lunch when going to work.

This will make it easier on the wallet over time. At some point, you will have to make a spreadsheet of all the money that you have saved by avoiding eating out. You can even prepare your own dinners and freeze them so you have lunch for several days at once. You'd be surprised how much money you'll save just from starting to do this.

46. Donate to charity organizations or projects in poor nations.

It may be surprising but there are so many great causes and ways in which you can help people all over the globe, whether it be financially, physically or just through some kind words of comfort during hard times. Not only will taking your time out to look at what's going on elsewhere teach you a lot about the world around you, but it will also help spread awareness and make everyone more aware of what's happening close by and elsewhere.

47. Go to a car-boot/second-hand market and buy something unusual you've always wanted but couldn't afford before.

Buy some retro items that might remind you of your childhood. The memories that may come with it will make you happy. Also, it's nice to remember the past sometimes and appreciate how far you have come.

48. Learn how to knit or sew.

Set it as a goal to make one item each week: from which you will create your own stockpile of knits, socks, scarves, and other goodies. You'll never know when such a hobby could come in handy. Even if you're not much of an artist, there are plenty of tutorials on the Internet that can get even the most novice beginner up and going in no time.

49. Learn to repurpose items for your own use.

You can save money by finding ways to reuse things you already have on hand, rather than buying new materials every time you need them. You're sure to find new uses for those old t-shirts you haven't worn since college that are just hanging in your closet or be thrilled at the idea of using some cardboard boxes to make bookends, storage bins, and other artful decor pieces.

50. Put up your own garage sale.

Have your own garage sale to make some extra money. Sell some of the old and unwanted things you have in your home; that CD collection, clothing that doesn't fit anymore, or those old broken appliances that just take up space in the basement. You can easily advertise these sales online by making flyers and posting them around town as well as on Craigslist and other popular public selling sites.

51. Watch an inspiring documentary with your friends or partner.

Find something that's uplifting and interesting to watch as a group. There are all sorts of documentary movies available about everything from scientific breakthroughs to historical events. It doesn't have to be boring or bland. Dig around for something really inspiring.

52. Find old cassette tapes and digitize them.

This can be a really fun and interesting project to do. You can create your own collections of classic songs. These song collections can be wonderful gifts to family and friends who love timeless music and melodies from the past.

53. Learn a new language online for free.

This may seem like a lofty goal, but it's totally possible to learn a new language for free. You can watch videos on YouTube and get the basics you need from there. After learning the basics for free, you can sign up with an online tutoring service that will really help hone your skills in a fun way.

54. Enroll in a yoga class.

The health and wellness benefits of yoga are endless. Not only will it help you physically but mentally too. Breathing, positive affirmations, and stretching can release endorphins that help with relieving yourself from the stress of feeling down or when depressed.

55. Find a painting or drawing class to take part in.

Art is a great way to express your feelings through colors and shapes. It also helps clear your mind and calm you down. It is said that people who take part in art classes are able to manage their emotions better and even have increased well-being.

56. Enroll in a self-defense class.

Something about kicking butt and protecting yourself can be hugely empowering. Feel-good hormones get released when your body is under stress so you'll be releasing endorphins as well. It also helps you to understand what types of things make you feel vulnerable as well as building your self-esteem.

57. Go fishing.

Fishing is considered an excellent stress reliever. Not only can you enjoy the process of fishing but you also get engaged on a more intellectual level, as well as nurture your mental health. Fishing requires a high level of concentration and awareness. This, like meditation, diverts your attention away from internal conflict and tension. As a result, it aids in the reduction of anxiety, the prevention of depression, and the promotion of relaxation. Moreover, fishing is also known to be a good workout for the upper body and back.

58. Sing alone.

In order to have fun, you don't need another person around you. Sing in front of a mirror, if you are too self-conscious about doing it in front of anyone else. Dance around your room with your favorite song playing on repeat, jumping as loudly as possible without any inhibition whatsoever. This is something that is best done when you are alone because everyone should do things their own way and enjoy things by themselves sometimes.

59. Take a bubble bath.

Fill a tub with warm water and add some bath bombs or use fresh flowers, herbs, or skin toning essential oils to make it more delightful. If desired, take along a bottle of wine and put on some relaxing music to create an even better atmosphere for self-care.

60. Get a pet.

It has been proven that pet owners have lower blood pressure, and are less likely to suffer from depression. People who take care of pets tend to live longer than those who don't. You can adopt one from an animal shelter. It's a great way to give back to your community while providing emotional support for yourself.

61. Memorize quotes.

Memorizing things may seem kind of useless at first glance, but psychologists say it's actually really good for building concentration and improving memory retention.

Memorizing quotes can be a really cool way to expand your library of knowledge on any particular subject.

62. Make a cup of tea when you get home from work.

You can also do this after doing another self-care activity. Tea has relaxing properties that help reduce mental fatigue and ease anxiety. You can try decaffeinated teas like mint, ginger, or lemon.

63. Eat some dark chocolate every day and don't feel guilty about it.

Chocolate can lower stress levels by lowering blood pressure and relaxing the nervous system. Dark chocolate gets an A+ rating on the Mood Meter scale from the University of Wisconsin-Madison's Health and Wellness Center because it's high in flavonoids, which are healthy compounds, and has little caffeine.

64. Get a manicure and pedicure.

When it's hot, you're going to sweat and it's gross. That's just a fact of life. But you don't have to sport those nasty-ass man hands. A well-maintained manicure makes your hands look smooth and sophisticated, like Ryan Gosling at a horse show or something. And, there's nothing more relaxing than getting a pedicure with some friends after work. You can choose to wear clear nail polish as a great way to make those nails clean and well-done.

65. Try aromatherapy.

Find an essential oil that works for you and either mix it into your soap or lotion. Or, try wearing a loose bracelet with powerful scents like lemon, vanilla, or peppermint. You can also try lighting an essential oil candle to create an ambiance that's good for relaxation.

66. Change your hair with a new hairstyle or haircut.

If you have short hair, grow it out a bit. If you've always wanted to try bangs, why not get them? If you have a full head of hair, why not go bald? Visit a barber or stylist and ask if they can shave your head for you. Get an undercut to make your hair appear shorter. Change the color of your hair by going blond or dark.

67. Get a facial or skincare treatment.

Men need this too as it will clean the pores left behind by shaving and help your skin appear healthy and vibrant. A facial can also help clear up pimples and acne, which is particularly beneficial for men who suffer from these common skin issues. Regardless of whether you have oily or dry skin, a facial can go a long way in cleaning your pores.

68. Moisturize regularly.

Many men neglect moisturizing and when they do, it is often just a simple lotion. Moisturizers are very important not only for the skin but also for helping to prevent breakouts as well. Try adding essential oils like lavender or tea tree oil to your lotions or creams and you can even try making your own.

69. Get your teeth cleaned.

It will make you feel better about yourself even if those hard and calcified structures found in the jaws don't need them yet. People will be more drawn to your smile too. You will also feel fresh and clean.

70. Go shopping for clothing.

Make the most of your wardrobe by adding some new items. Get new underwear, socks, and undershirts to replenish what you already have. Pick up a new button-down shirt for the office. Choose a few new pairs of jeans that fit you well. Go shopping for some tank tops and t-shirts to wear when it's warm outside.

71. Declutter your living area or bedroom with organizing tips.

Remove everything from your closets and drawers so you can organize them more effectively. If your closet is very small, group similar items together to maximize space. For instance, all shirts go on one side of the rod. Remove any unwanted clothing from your bedroom and other areas in the house where they are not needed.

72. Visit a place from memory where positive memories were made.

This place could be one that evokes fondness and happiness even if it was a long time ago. This could be a park or playground where you played as a child, maybe on the swingset or slide. Or perhaps, this was your first school classroom; the tree in front of your house when you were little; an open field near water, such as a creek or lake, where you played as a child.

73. Plan a day at an art gallery or craft museum.

If you have an interest in art or craftsmanship, plan a day trip to the nearest art gallery or craft museum. Spend the day exploring different displays of artwork. You might even contact the museum and see if they have openings for volunteers.

74. Plan a trip to an amusement or water park.

Plan a trip with your family or friends to the local water park or amusement park. Take a picnic lunch so you can save money. Perhaps, you can stick around for dinner and a few hours of nighttime entertainment.

75. Attend shows at theaters, like plays and improv comedy performances.

This is a fun and inexpensive activity that you or your whole family will enjoy. The activity will be more interesting if you all dress up like the characters in your favorite play or movie. Just make sure to get tickets in advance.

76. Visit botanical gardens and zoos in your area.

Both of these venues have beautiful flowers and animals, in addition to being budget-friendly. Sometimes zoos will even have "free days" or special family-friendly events where admission is greatly reduced. Find out what is a short drive away and plan to make a day of visiting all the sights.

77. Play word or logic games in the park.

This is a great thing to do with friends that you want to get to know more. Bring a laptop, smartphone, or tablet, and enjoy the time outdoors while you make new friends. While you're at it, you may bring some snacks too.

78. Go to a house of worship.

You may go to a church, synagogue, any house of worship depending on your religion. With this, you may be able to feel that sense of community by praying together with others. Having a strong support system is very important in dealing with stress.

79. Play a musical instrument.

It is amazing how good you will feel when you play an instrument, whether you can play well or not. Play it as loud as possible. If you do not have a musical instrument, borrow one from a friend. Be creative and let go of those inhibitions. For sure, you will feel so much better after you play.

80. Try writing down some lyrics and singing them into an audio recorder.

You may even send an email with the song attached to all your family members. Include pictures if possible. It's great fun for everyone involved and they will appreciate the time that was taken to create something special just for them. Follow up with a phone call the same day— even if you just leave a voice message and sing a part of the song you have created for them.

81. Write about what's bothering you in a letter.

You don't have to mail it. You may tear up the paper so that no one else sees the words. This helps get out your bottled feelings without hurting anyone else or yourself by saying things you may regret later or even doing something foolish like getting into a fight with someone who doesn't deserve fighting with.

82. Volunteer at a local soup kitchen or homeless shelter.

Doing this may make you feel more humble. When you help others, it helps you appreciate what you have even more. It is something that you can do without spending money, and you will be learning about giving back while having fun.

83. Let your dog sleep with you at night.

They will provide more joy than any old pillow ever could. They will make it so much easier for you to fall asleep and they can hear "your heartbeat," which is very relaxing for pets.

84. If you have a backyard, invite over your friends and family for a game of soccer or football.

Get some cones to mark the goals so that there is no confusion about how big or small they should be. Any outdoor sport is great but this one really brings out the competitive spirit in people. You can have teams or make it fun for everyone by just having a non-competitive game.

85. Jump up and down on that cold tile floor in bare feet.

This increases circulation which helps deliver fresh oxygen and nutrients to every cell in your body. Plus, it's good exercise. Try not to think how silly you look jumping around by yourself and just smile! The faster the better.

86. Take pictures of beautiful spots.

Get your camera or camera phone out every day and take a picture of something you find beautiful. It could be the sky, a sunset or a tree in blossom. Then, make these into a collage at the end of the year and enjoy.

87. Go for a drive in the country.

Find somewhere faraway where you can watch the sunset uninterrupted. The colors will differentiate themselves as they merge together. And by daybreak, everything will seem new again.

88. Travel to somewhere exotic.

This helps you get out of your normal routine and forces you to do new things. You can choose a place that enables you to be in contact with nature or somewhere adventurous. It may be something local that you have never been to or it could be an international trip. Either way, it's worth a shot.

89. Read an inspiring book.

Choose a book that inspires you, that gives you a sense of passion and purpose. You could also read some biographies to encourage your own ambition. This will also help you to focus on the good things in life and make you significantly happier.

90. Start listening to podcasts while you drive.

This will keep your mind stimulated and learning new stuff is always fun. Just be selective about what kind of content they are; otherwise, this could just lead to more stress if it's upsetting stuff. There are some great podcasts out there with inspiring people that are perfect for de-stressing.

91. Watch funny Youtube videos.

Watching funny videos is great because it allows your mind to "switch off" and laugh for a while. The best part about watching comedy is that you don't even have to think. Your brain automatically reacts and thinks about the story or jokes, which helps you let go of some stress while watching these videos. This will also make you feel good and positive which is another big aspect of self-care.

92. Read a comic book that you haven't read in years.

If you find old comic books that you used to read as a child or teenager, try reading them again. You will probably be surprised by how much you have forgotten and how much you enjoyed things that your older self didn't think too highly of.

93. Do random acts of kindness for strangers.

Perhaps, you can pay for someone's coffee or lunch. Or you may hold open a door for someone behind you. You will feel amazing and it will help you to connect with people in a more positive way.

94. Write a story.

Whether it's a personal story in your life or a fictional one about characters from another world, writing stories can keep your mind active as well as help relieve tension from stressful situations in your own life. The greatest thing about writing though is that if there are things bothering you, then venting them out in fiction will help improve your mood as well as your creativity.

95. Start doing vlogs.

Some people think that it takes a lot of effort to do videos but actually, this can be one of the more fun things you will ever experience. If you have a camera and plan on making vlogs, then go for it. You'll realize how easy they are once you get started. The amount of creativity that vlogs can bring into your life is endless. You have complete liberty to do whatever you want in front of your camera.

96. Write in a journal.

Write down all the things in your life that are making you happy and satisfied. Think about where these feelings come from and write them down too. This can be very therapeutic because you often get so caught up in life that you forget to focus on what makes you happy.

97. Take some time out from technology.

Make sure that at least one day in a week, you switch off your phone, computer, and social media so you can spend time being present with yourself instead of being buried in the screen. If it's difficult, start small by switching all this stuff off in the evening before bedtime so there are no distractions when you're winding down.

98. Write a prayer.

You don't have to be super religious but writing down all your worries and putting them into a prayer works really well. Nowadays, people have become so obsessed with phones and gadgets, it's much harder to remember the good things, so this activity will help you out massively, especially with embracing your spirituality.

99. Make a list of all the people in your life that care about, love, and support you.

Make sure to contact each one by phone or email and let them know how much they mean to you. This will help you to feel more connected to others and less isolated. Make time for them personally too. Give someone a call or visit them. Perhaps, go out for coffee together or do something fun.

100. Get enough sleep.

It is vital to get enough sleep otherwise your body and your brain won't function properly. Sleep is very important for everyone, especially for men trying to gain muscles. First of all, sleep regulates your body's hormones that play a big role in muscle building. Secondly, you will have more time to exercise if you go to bed early and wake up early enough. Third, you will be physically and mentally refreshed when you need it the most. Get at least 7 hours of sleep every night, if possible.

Conclusion

It is no secret that men often put themselves last on the list of priorities. The idea of self-care is even met with some resistance for many, who feel they should be tough and take care of others before themselves. But, with the amount of roles men play in society—spouse, father, boss, employee, and friend, among them—there's not a lot of time left that can be devoted to oneself.

In these times, it is hard to make time for self-care or prioritize the importance of relaxing activities. But, whether you're an entrepreneur, health care staff, technology worker, or just someone who feels you have too much on your plate, making time for yourself is more important than ever.

I know how busy you are, and I'm glad that I was able to share with you some amazing tips and activities on how to take care of yourself. Our bodies are designed to feel relaxed and comfortable when it experiences stress. That's why you need to avoid stressful situations. It is not just because they are uncomfortable—it is because they can actually make you physically sick in the process. Fortunately, there are ways you can take steps to reduce your stress levels so that you feel more refreshed. And those activities don't have to cost a ton of money or time. Many people get great results from simple exercises they can do at home or during their lunch break. There is no right way for how long these activities should be performed, but most experts believe shorter bursts of activities are best for helping ease stress over the long term.

Certainly, it can be beneficial to have a self-care routine that incorporates tools or activities intended to foster the wellness of the mind, body, and soul. Similarly, there is no need for men to feel shame about taking time out of their day to do things like going for a walk in nature or sitting down to meditate.

These self-care activities for men have helped a variety of individuals relax or recharge, and they can work just as well if you give them a chance to become part of your routine. You might enjoy doing these activities that can help you become less tired and anxious. With these routines, you can better focus on the things that are most important in life. Or maybe it will inspire you to try something completely different.

Looking after yourself will only allow you to do more for your loved ones, so it shouldn't be ignored or denied. By giving yourself the chance to relax and unwind or nurture your mind and body, you will be able to come back refreshed and ready for anything that comes up in your day-to-day life.

Leaving a Review

As an independent author with limited marketing resources, reviews for my books are essential in order to survive as an indie writer. New works of literature get published daily, so there's no guarantee that any given work will be successful.

Your review can help authors like me grow and share their knowledge with more people. If you enjoyed this book, I would really appreciate your honest feedback. You can leave a review by going to this book's page on Amazon, where it is listed, and clicking "Write A Review."

Leaving an honest review can also help other people find this book easily on Amazon and benefit from it as well. Your feedback is important to me so I can find out what you like and don't, which in turn helps me make better decisions about my writing style.

Thank you,

Edgar